Artificial Intelligence (AI) And Healthcare: The Promise And Threats Of AI In Medicine

Peterson Walkers

Table of contents

Introduction

Part I

Part II

Part III

Conclusion

Introduction

- AI and healthcare: the current landscape
- Overview of the promises and threats of AI in healthcare

Healthcare is not an exception to how artificial intelligence (AI) is changing many different sectors. Healthcare providers are increasingly turning to AI as a way to improve patient outcomes, save costs, and raise overall standards of care.

The use of AI in healthcare nowadays has many different applications. Medical imaging is one of the most frequently used applications of AI in healthcare. To analyze medical pictures like X-rays, CT scans, and MRIs, AI algorithms are being created and trained. Medical personnel may discover and diagnose problems like cancer or fractures more quickly and precisely by utilizing AI.

Drug development is another area of healthcare where AI is being applied. Compared to conventional approaches, AI systems may find new medication candidates more rapidly and precisely. This might quicken the discovery of new drugs that could save the lives of individuals with critical diseases.

AI is also being used in healthcare to save costs and enhance patient outcomes. Predictive analytics, for instance, may be used to identify people who are highly likely to develop a certain medical condition, enabling healthcare professionals to take early action and stop the problem from forming or worsening. AI may also be utilized to streamline hospital operations and enhance resource management, resulting in lower costs and more effectiveness.

Despite these advantages, there are reservations regarding the application of AI in healthcare. The possibility of prejudice and discrimination is one of the main worries. AI algorithms may reinforce and magnify biases already present in the healthcare system if they are not created and trained using diverse information. Furthermore, there are worries about patient security and privacy because AI algorithms might be trained using private patient information.

In summary, the present state of AI in healthcare is complicated, having both advantages and disadvantages. While AI has the potential to revolutionize healthcare by enhancing patient outcomes and lowering costs, it is crucial to use it responsibly and with caution. We can make sure AI is utilized in a manner that helps patients and healthcare professionals by addressing issues like prejudice and privacy.

By boosting overall care quality, lowering healthcare costs, and improving patient outcomes, artificial intelligence (AI) has the potential to completely transform the healthcare industry. The employment of AI in healthcare is, however, not without serious risks and difficulties.

The capacity of AI to increase the precision and speed of medical diagnostics is one of the major promises it holds for the future of healthcare. To find trends and arrive at more precise diagnoses, AI systems may examine vast volumes of medical data, including patient histories, test findings, and medical pictures. This may result in earlier illness identification and more efficient therapies, which will benefit patients' outcomes and quality of life.

AI can also speed up the creation of new drugs, which might save the lives of people with critical ailments. AI has the potential to drastically shorten the time and expense associated with bringing new pharmaceuticals to market by finding prospective drug candidates more rapidly and accurately than conventional techniques.

AI can also assist streamline hospital processes and enhance resource allocation, which will save costs and increase efficiency. Healthcare practitioners may intervene early and stop an illness from forming or worsening by using predictive analytics to identify individuals who are at a high risk of getting a certain medical condition.

Despite these benefits, using AI in healthcare is also fraught with serious risks and difficulties. The potential for prejudice and discrimination is a danger. AI algorithms may reinforce and magnify biases already present in the healthcare system if they are not created and trained using diverse information. This could lead to discrepancies in patient outcomes and uneven access to healthcare.

The possibility of privacy and security breaches is another danger. Sensitive patient data may be used to train AI systems, putting the data at risk of theft or abuse. Furthermore, there are issues with the lack of accountability and transparency in AI decision-making, as well as the possibility of errors and misdiagnosis.

In conclusion, AI has great promise for healthcare, with the ability to increase the overall quality of treatment, lower costs, and improve patient outcomes. To guarantee that AI is utilized in a manner that helps patients and healthcare professionals, it is crucial to approach the use of AI in healthcare with caution and responsibility, addressing issues like bias, privacy, and accountability.

Part I: Promises

Precision medicine: how AI is helping to tailor treatments to individual patients

Healthcare is not an exception to how artificial intelligence (AI) is transforming many different sectors. Personalized medicine, a fast-expanding area that customizes therapies for individual patients based on their unique genetic composition, lifestyle, and environment, has been made possible by the introduction of AI in medicine. This strategy represents a substantial divergence from the conventional one-size-fits-all approach, which often yields unfavorable outcomes and unneeded side effects. Personalized medicine is positioned to provide the best treatment results, save healthcare costs, and increase patient happiness by using AI.

The analysis of enormous volumes of data is one of the main ways AI is allowing customized treatment. Understanding the complicated interactions between genes, proteins, and other biological components in the enormously complex system that is the human body is a difficult undertaking. Massive datasets may be sorted through AI algorithms, which can then spot relationships and patterns that are invisible to people. This skill enables scientists to get a fresh understanding of the underlying causes of illnesses and create focused treatments that cater to the unique requirements of each patient.

AI has helped us comprehend diseases like cancer, which are characterized by the unchecked development of aberrant cells, for instance. Rather than being a single illness, cancer is a collection of more than 100 distinct forms, each with a distinctive genetic profile. AI systems can discover the precise mutations fueling the development of cancer cells and forecast which therapies are most likely to be beneficial for each patient by examining the genetic data of thousands of cancer patients. With the use of this tailored strategy, numerous ground-breaking medicines have already been created, including the use of immune checkpoint inhibitors to treat certain forms of lung cancer and melanoma.

The creation of new drugs is another area where AI is having a big influence. A new drug's introduction to the market is often a lengthy, costly, and high-failure procedure. However, by identifying which compounds are most likely to be effective against a specific target, AI can speed up this process and significantly cut the time and money needed for drug development. The chance of success may be further increased by using AI to assist in identifying possible side effects and safety issues early in the research process.

Precision diagnostics are critical for individualized treatment, and AI is playing a significant role in their development. AI algorithms may find biomarkers that signal the existence of a certain illness or forecast the possibility of acquiring a particular ailment by examining a patient's genetic data. With the use of this knowledge, diagnostic tests may be created that are both highly accurate and less intrusive, allowing for early diagnosis and intervention.

Additionally, mobile apps and wearable technology powered by AI are assisting patients in keeping track of their health and making educated decisions about their treatment. These gadgets may monitor vital signs, examine sleep patterns, and provide individualized dietary and exercise advice, all of which improve health results.

Personalized medicine has enormous promise, but there are also obstacles to be addressed. A major challenge is ensuring the security and privacy of sensitive patient data, as well as the need for standardized and compatible data formats. In addition, further study is required to comprehend the moral ramifications of AI-driven healthcare decision-making.

Diagnosis: how AI is improving the accuracy and speed of medical diagnoses

The use of artificial intelligence (AI) in medical diagnostics has been one of the most important recent developments in the rapidly changing area of healthcare. The precision and speed of identifying a wide range of medical illnesses, from everyday aches and pains to life-threatening diseases, is being revolutionized by AI algorithms and machine learning approaches. This area examines how AI is reshaping healthcare by enhancing patient outcomes, altering the diagnosis process, and more.

Increasing Diagnostic Precision
Accurate medical diagnosis is essential for efficient treatment and patient care. Systems driven by AI have shown to be very effective in increasing diagnostic precision. AI algorithms can find patterns and abnormalities in a massive quantity of

medical data, including patient records, photographs, and research articles, that may not be immediately obvious to human doctors.

Medical imaging analysis is one of the areas where AI has shown promising outcomes. Convolutional Neural Networks (CNNs), a subset of deep learning algorithms, have been used to accurately analyze mammograms, CT images, and X-rays. These artificial intelligence (AI) systems can recognize minor abnormalities, early-stage cancers, and other irregularities, allowing for earlier treatment and better patient outcomes.

Increasing the Diagnostic Process' Speed
When it comes to making a medical diagnosis, time is often important. Increased medical expenses, worse conditions, and long-suffering may all result from delayed or protracted diagnosis. The time needed to provide an accurate

diagnosis is being drastically cut down thanks to AI technology.

In-the-moment meaningful insights and suggestions may be given to healthcare workers by AI algorithms that can swiftly process and evaluate large volumes of patient data, medical literature, and clinical guidelines. AI technologies allow doctors to concentrate more on patient care by automating time-consuming chores like data input, analysis, and cross-referencing. This eventually results in quicker diagnosis and prompt treatment.

Making Clinical Decisions with Support
For healthcare practitioners, AI-powered diagnostic tools serve as trustworthy decision support systems. These technologies help doctors make better-informed judgments by offering crucial second perspectives. AI algorithms may provide differential diagnoses, recommend suitable testing, and offer

treatment regimens based on evidence-based recommendations by examining the patient's symptoms, medical history, and test findings.

Additionally, AI-driven diagnostic tools continuously learn from fresh information and clinical experiences, enhancing their precision and expertise over time. The best possible patient care is made possible by this iterative learning process, which guarantees that doctors have access to the most recent developments in medical research and diagnostics.

Challenges and Long-Term Effects
While AI has enormous potential to increase diagnostic speed and accuracy, there are still several obstacles that need to be overcome before it can be widely used. Critical factors in the integration of AI in healthcare include ensuring data privacy and security, correcting biases in AI systems, and retaining openness in decision-making.

A successful adoption also requires educating healthcare workers on how to use AI technologies and smoothly integrating AI into current processes.

Looking forward, artificial intelligence will continue to be crucial to medical diagnosis. As technology develops, AI algorithms will grow more advanced, capable of deciphering complicated data and making more precise predictions about the course of diseases. The accuracy and timeliness of medical diagnosis will be further improved by integrating AI with other diagnostic techniques, such as wearable technology and genetic testing.

Early detection: how AI is helping to catch diseases early when they are more treatable

Long-term patient outcomes are significantly improved by early illness identification. Early diagnosis of an illness typically makes it more durable and increases the likelihood that it will be cured. Unfortunately, early disease detection is frequently difficult, and many people do not receive a diagnosis until their condition has advanced to a more serious stage. But early disease detection is now more conceivable thanks to artificial intelligence (AI) technology, and patients could benefit greatly from this.

The field of medicine is being quickly transformed by AI, and early detection is one application that has shown significant promise. Huge volumes of medical data may be analyzed by AI algorithms, which can also spot patterns and connections and provide insights that human practitioners would overlook. The application of AI to enhance early illness diagnosis across a variety of medical problems will be discussed in this article.

Cancer Screening

Finding the illness early on is one of the biggest obstacles to effective cancer therapy. Early cancer detection greatly increases the likelihood of effective therapy. However, because the symptoms are subtle and the disease may not yet be visible on imaging tests, early-stage cancers are frequently challenging to identify. By looking for indicators of disease in medical imaging like lung scans and mammograms, AI is being used to increase the accuracy of cancer diagnosis. Artificial intelligence (AI) systems may spot small tissue changes that human radiologists would overlook, decreasing false negatives and boosting the chance of early diagnosis.

Detection of Cardiovascular Disease

The most common cause of mortality globally is cardiovascular disease (CVD), and avoiding heart attacks and strokes depends on early identification.

By examining information from electrocardiograms (ECGs) and other cardiac monitoring devices, AI is being utilized to increase the accuracy of CVD identification. AI algorithms can detect small variations in heart function that might be a sign of CVD in its early stages. Early detection of these alterations enables patients to obtain medication and lifestyle adjustments that may halt or even stop the disease's development.

Detection of Infectious Diseases
The crucial value of early infectious illness diagnosis has been brought to light by the COVID-19 pandemic. AI has been crucial in the development of diagnostic testing and epidemic prediction. For instance, AI algorithms have been used to examine medical photographs of the lungs of COVID-19 patients and find the disease's

early warning symptoms. Additionally, AI is being used to create predictive models that can forecast the spread of infectious diseases and guide public health interventions.

Moral and legal issues to consider

Although AI shows great promise for detecting diseases early, it also raises significant ethical and legal questions. For instance, there are worries regarding the security of patient data and privacy, as well as the possibility that AI algorithms would perpetuate current prejudices in healthcare. When an AI system makes a mistaken diagnosis, there is also the issue of culpability. It is crucial to create rules and policies that address these challenges and make sure AI is utilized safely and morally as it becomes more commonplace in healthcare.

The Future of AI in Detecting Early Disease

The use of AI in the early diagnosis of diseases has enormous promise, and in the years to come, the technology is anticipated to advance further. Widespread adoption is, however, nevertheless hampered by fundamental obstacles, such as the high cost of AI technology and the need for expensive infrastructure and training. However, AI will likely become a more important tool in early disease detection and better patient outcomes as the technology becomes more widely available.

Drug discovery: how AI is accelerating the development of new medications

Despite these difficulties, AI's role in drug discovery has a promising future. Artificial intelligence (AI) is projected to become a more crucial tool for medication research as technology progresses. Better patient outcomes and the development of more efficient therapies may follow from this.

How AI is enhancing the interpretation of medical pictures in imaging for medicine

X-rays, CT scans, and MRIs are just a few examples of the types of medical imaging that are vital to the diagnosis and treatment of many illnesses. However, analyzing medical images can take some time and requires specialists with extensive training. Medical imaging analysis is undergoing a revolution as a result of the development of artificial intelligence (AI) technologies. In this post, we'll look at how AI is being

used to enhance medical picture processing and the potential advantages for patients.

Medical Image Analysis Using AI
Medical personnel may identify and treat patients with increased precision and speed because of AI algorithms' quick and accurate analysis of medical imagery. AI may be used, for instance, to spot patterns and irregularities in medical imaging that may be hard for the human eye to see.

Machine learning is one sort of AI algorithm utilized in the study of medical imaging. By examining massive datasets of annotated photos, machine learning algorithms may be taught to spot patterns in medical images. These algorithms can reliably spot patterns and abnormalities in fresh photos after being taught, negating the need for human examination.

Deep learning is a different kind of AI algorithm utilized in the study of medical imaging. To identify intricate patterns in pictures, such as the size and structure of organs or the presence of malignancies, deep learning algorithms are used. Deep learning algorithms can precisely find patterns and abnormalities that human analysts may overlook by examining vast databases of medical photos.

AI's Advantages in medical image analysis
There are various possible advantages of using AI for medical image analysis. First, it may considerably cut down on the time and expense involved in interpreting medical pictures. Medical personnel may spend more time providing patient care and less time reviewing photos by automating the analysis process.

Second, AI may aid medical practitioners in choosing treatments and diagnoses that are more accurate. AI systems may uncover patterns and abnormalities in medical photos that would be difficult for the human eye to see by processing them more quickly and accurately. This may therefore result in improved patient outcomes and therapeutic efficacy.

The lack of qualified medical practitioners in certain locations may also be helped by AI. AI algorithms may lessen the requirement for highly skilled medical experts to interpret medical pictures by automating the analysis process. This may make healthcare more accessible in places with few medical resources.

AI in Medical Imaging Analysis Examples
Today, there are many instances of AI being used in medical image analysis. A deep learning system, for instance, was employed by researchers at the Massachusetts Institute of Technology (MIT) to scan mammograms and find patterns that could

suggest breast cancer. The computer was able to detect breast cancer in more freshin more fresh pictures than human radiologists after being trained on a dataset of over 60,000 mammograms.

Another example is the employment of AI to examine brain MRIs. A deep learning system was utilized by University of California, San Francisco researchers to examine the MRI scans of Alzheimer's patients. Up to six years before the onset of clinical signs, the algorithm was able to correctly identify which individuals will eventually acquire Alzheimer's disease.

Analysis of the Problems and Future of AI in Medical Imaging
While AI has a lot of potential for medical image analysis, there are also many obstacles to overcome. For instance, there are worries regarding the precision of AI algorithms and the possibility of bias in the training sets of data. In addition, ethical

issues including patient confidentiality and data security must be taken into account.

The future of AI in medical imaging analysis is promising despite these difficulties. AI is likely to become an increasingly important tool for medical professionals as technology progresses. In turn, this might lead to more precise diagnoses, wiser medical choices, and better patient outcomes.

AI is transforming.

Part II: Threats

Bias and discrimination. how AI can perpetuate and amplify biases in healthcare

To improve patient outcomes and increase the effectiveness of healthcare delivery, artificial intelligence (AI) is being employed more and more in the industry. However, there are worries that AI could exacerbate and perpetuate existing biases in the medical field, resulting in discrimination and unequal access to care.

In this post, we'll look at how prejudice and discrimination in the healthcare industry may be strengthened and perpetuated, as well as what steps can be taken to reduce these hazards.

How AI Maintains and Strengthens Discrimination and Bias

The data that AI systems are educated on determines how objective they are. Healthcare biases will continue and become more pronounced if the data used to train an AI machine is prejudiced. For instance, an AI program may be less accurate at identifying medical diseases among patients of color if it was trained on data that mostly represented white people.

Through feedback loops, AI can also reinforce and amplify prejudices. It is possible to feed biased outputs from an AI algorithm back into the system, which would reinforce and exacerbate the biases. This might lead to a vicious cycle of prejudice that is hard to stop.

Healthcare AI bias and discrimination examples;

There are several instances in which prejudice and discrimination are strengthened by AI in the healthcare industry. For instance, a study conducted by researchers at Stanford University discovered that a skin cancer detection AI system performed worse when detecting skin lesions in individuals with darker skin tones. The algorithm's findings are biased since it was developed on a sample of patients who were mostly light-skinned.

Using AI algorithms to detect people who are at high risk of acquiring chronic medical issues is another example. Patients from underprivileged backgrounds may be discriminated against by these algorithms since they may have less access to resources like healthcare and other tools that might lower their chance of acquiring chronic diseases.

Questions and Answers

Several obstacles need to be overcome to address bias and discrimination in healthcare AI. The lack of variety in the data used to train AI systems is one of the major problems. AI algorithms should be trained on datasets that are representative of the population they will be used to serve to lower the risk of bias. Additional data from underrepresented populations may be needed to address this.

The need to create and apply ethical guidelines for the use of AI in healthcare presents another difficulty. These guidelines should include topics like data privacy, accountability, and openness. An emphasis should also be placed on ensuring that AI is utilized in healthcare to support, not replace, human decision-making.

Privacy and Security: How AI compromises patient data security and Privacy

By boosting patient outcomes and the effectivencoo of hcalthcaro dolivory, artificial intelligence (AI) has the potential to change the industry. However, as the application of AI in healthcare grows, so do worries about patient data security and privacy. This area will examine the concerns AI presents to patient data security and privacy, as well as what can be done to reduce such risks.

Security Risks

The possibility of data breaches is one of the primary privacy hazards connected to AI in healthcare. To be taught efficiently, AI systems need a lot of data, some of which may include patients' sensitive personal information. A breach of patient privacy might occur if this data is not securely safeguarded against unauthorized access.

The possibility of data abuse is another privacy danger. AI algorithms may unearth previously undisclosed facts about patients, which might be utilized for immoral things like insurance discrimination or targeted advertising.

Security dangers

AI in healthcare has security problems in addition to privacy risks. To acquire patient data that might be used for identity theft or other illegal activities, hackers may try to compromise healthcare networks. Hackers may also attack AI algorithms to fool them into producing inaccurate findings.

The possibility for AI systems to make mistakes is another security danger. The safety and health of patients might be seriously impacted if an AI program yields erroneous findings. For instance, if a medical diagnosis algorithm returns a false negative, a patient could not get the care they need, which might make their situation worse.

Reducing Risks

Various things may be done to reduce the hazards that come with AI in healthcare. Making sure that patient data is adequately safeguarded is among the most crucial things. This includes security precautions like network segmentation, access controls, and encryption. Healthcare firms should also make sure that all of their staff members have received the necessary training on data privacy and security best practices.

The implementation of ethical guidelines for the use of AI in healthcare is a crucial next step. These guidelines should include topics like data privacy, accountability, and openness. For patients to understand how and why their data is being utilized, there should also be an emphasis on ensuring that AI algorithms are transparent in their decision-making processes.

Errors and incorrect diagnosis: How AI may hurt people

Because it can help with the diagnosis and treatment of a wide range of medical conditions, artificial intelligence (AI) is becoming a more and more common tool in the healthcare industry. However, AI systems are not perfect, and they occasionally commit errors that endanger patients. We will examine possible hazards related to applying AI to healthcare in this post, along with mitigation strategies.

Potential dangers

The possibility of incorrect diagnosis is one of the key dangers connected to the use of AI in healthcare. Large datasets that may not always be complete or representative of the patient population are used to train AI systems. As a consequence, they can diagnose patients incorrectly or overlook crucial information, which might result in improper or delayed therapy.

The possibility for AI systems to make mistakes is another possible issue. For the safety and health of patients, it may have major repercussions if an AI system generates erroneous findings. For instance, if a medical diagnosis algorithm returns a false negative, a patient could not get the care they need, which might make their situation worse.

Reducing Risks

Several steps can be taken to reduce the risks connected with using AI in healthcare. Making suresure AI algorithms are clear in their decision-making processes is one of the most crucial things to do. This implies that healthcare professionals need to have a thorough grasp of how the algorithms operate, the types of data they are trained on, and any possible biases or limits in the algorithms.

Making suresure healthcare professionals have the necessary skills and knowledge to appropriately evaluate and apply AI-generated outcomes is another crucial step. Understanding AI system limits and incorporating AI-generated data into healthcare decision-making processes are part of this.

Last but not least, it's critical to make sure AI systems are continually assessed and monitored to spot and correct any faults or biases that may manifest. This may be achieved by continuously validating AI algorithms and testing them, as well as by using feedback systems that let healthcare professionals report any problems or concerns with AI-generated findings.

Although AI has the potential to increase healthcare delivery's precision and effectiveness, it is not a perfect solution and occasionally makes mistakes that put patients at risk. Healthcare providers must take precautions to guarantee that AI algorithms are open and understandable, that staff members are properly trained and skilled in the interpretation and application of results generated by AI, and that AI systems are continuously assessed and monitored to spot and correct any biases or errors. By doing this, we can make sure that AI is utilized in healthcare ethically and responsibly, which will eventually improve patient outcomes.

AI raises concerns about who is ultimately accountable for making medical choices in terms of transparency and accountability.

The growing use of artificial intelligence (AI) in healthcare is posing significant problems concerning accountability and transparency. When AI is engaged, who is in charge of making medical decisions? How can we guarantee that AI algorithms are responsible for their acts and that their decision-making processes are transparent?

AI's Place in Healthcare

By increasing the precision and effectiveness of medical diagnosis and treatments, AI has the potential to completely transform healthcare. AI systems can find patterns and links in vast volumes of data that may not be immediately obvious to human therapists. Better patient outcomes, quicker diagnosis, and more individualized treatment regimens may result from this.

But there are also significant ethical concerns about accountability and transparency raised by the use of AI in healthcare. AI algorithms are unable to clearly explain their decision-making processes to people in the same way that human physicians can. This might make it challenging for patients and healthcare professionals to comprehend the processes involved in making medical choices as well as who is ultimately in charge of them.

AI Decision-Making Transparency

It's crucial to guarantee that AI algorithms are open about how they make decisions to allay these worries. This implies that healthcare professionals need to have a thorough grasp of how the algorithms operate, the types of data they are trained on, and any possible biases or limits in the algorithms.

Using explainable AI (XAI) methods is one approach to attain transparency. Healthcare professionals may follow an AI algorithm's decision-making process using XAI techniques, which makes it simpler to grasp how the algorithm came to a given result. This may assist to increase confidence in AI-generated findings and make sure that patients and healthcare professionals are satisfied with the choices being made.

Taking Responsibility for AI Decisions

It's crucial to make sure that AI algorithms are responsible for their behaviors in addition to being transparent. This may be difficult since AI algorithms can't be held accountable for their choices the same way that people can.

Making AI algorithm creators and users accountable for their behavior is one possible answer. This implies that any unfavorable effects of using AI systems should be the responsibility of the businesses and organizations that create and implement such systems.

Another strategy is to create rules and laws that guarantee the moral and responsible use of AI in healthcare. This may include rules for the creation and use of AI algorithms as well as rules for the appropriate application of AI-generated outcomes in clinical decision-making procedures.

AI is integrating more and more into healthcare, which is posing crucial queries regarding accountability and transparency. It is crucial to make sure AI algorithms are transparent in their decision-making processes and that they are held responsible for their acts to guarantee that AI is utilized ethically and responsibly. This may be accomplished by using XAI methodologies, rules, and guidelines and by making AI algorithm creators and operators accountable for their deeds. We can make sure AI is used in a manner that helps patients and society as a whole if we do this.

Part III: Ethics and Governance

How to guarantee that AI is utilized in healthcare morally and responsibly are ethical factors

It is vital to make sure that artificial intelligence (AI) is utilized in healthcare ethically and responsibly as it continues to be incorporated into the industry. By increasing the precision and effectiveness of medical diagnosis and treatments, AI has the potential to completely transform healthcare. It also brings up significant ethical issues around responsibility, prejudice, and data privacy.

Data Security
Data privacy is a crucial ethical issue when using AI in healthcare. To learn and produce reliable predictions, AI systems need a lot of

data. To safeguard patient privacy, this data must be used with caution, however.

Healthcare providers should adhere to established data privacy laws, such as the Health Insurance Portability and Accountability Act (HIPAA) in the United States, to guarantee data privacy. To prevent unauthorized access to or exploitation of patient data, healthcare providers should also have strong data security safeguards in place.

Bias
Bias is a further ethical issue to be taken into account when using AI in healthcare. The quality of AI algorithms depends on the data they are trained on. The algorithms will be biased if the data is skewed.

Healthcare professionals should make sure that the data used to train the algorithms is varied and representative of the patient population to combat bias in AI. To find and eliminate any potential bias, healthcare practitioners should routinely assess the effectiveness of AI algorithms.

Accountability

Last but not least, accountability is a crucial ethical factor to take into account when using AI in healthcare. Making sure that the accountable parties are held accountable for their actions is crucial as AI algorithms are increasingly used in healthcare decision-making.

Healthcare professionals must be open and honest about how AI is used in clinical judgment. Patients ought to be made aware of the use of AI and given the chance to give their informed consent. Furthermore, the accuracy and effectiveness of AI systems should be the responsibility of the developers and operators of the algorithms.

It is crucial to think about the ethical implications of AI use as it is more and more integrated into healthcare. To ensure that AI is used ethically and responsibly, ethical issues like data privacy, bias, and accountability must be addressed. The use of AI by healthcare practitioners must be disclosed, and the creators and operators of AI algorithms must be held responsible for their activities. We can make sure that AI is utilized to enhance patient outcomes while respecting the strictest ethical guidelines by taking these ethical issues into account.

Regulatory challenges: how to guarantee the safety and effectiveness of AI in healthcare

By increasing the precision and effectiveness of medical diagnosis and treatments, the incorporation of artificial intelligence (AI) into healthcare has the potential to completely transform the sector. It also presents substantial regulatory difficulties, however. Regulators must deal with problems like safety, effectiveness, and transparency if they want to make sure AI is safe and useful in healthcare.

Safety
Safety is one of the most important regulatory problems facing the use of AI in healthcare. The quality of AI algorithms depends on the data they are trained on. The algorithms may decide inadvertently, harming patients, if the data is flawed or prejudiced. Furthermore, AI algorithms can

make errors that would not be made by actual medical professionals.

Regulators must demand that AI algorithms be fully vetted and verified before they are utilized in clinical settings to address these safety issues. Additionally, regulators must set forth specific rules for the application of AI algorithms in the healthcare industry and hold healthcare providers liable for adhering to those rules.

Efficacy
Efficacy is a different regulatory obstacle when using AI in healthcare. AI algorithms must be successful in enhancing patient outcomes to be useful. To make sure AI algorithms are successful in enhancing health outcomes, regulators must mandate that they be thoroughly examined.

Transparency

Finally, transparency is an essential regulatory challenge in the use of AI in healthcare. Patients must have confidence in the safety and efficacy of AI algorithms. Patients may find it difficult to assess the effectiveness and complexity of AI algorithms since they are often sophisticated.

Regulators must demand that healthcare providers disclose the use of AI algorithms in medical decision-making to address this problem. When AI is employed, patients must be informed, and healthcare professionals must be able to explain how the AI algorithms function and how they are used to make medical choices.

To guarantee AI's effectiveness and safety, authorities must solve important regulatory hurdles as AI continues to be incorporated into healthcare. Among the regulatory difficulties that must be solved are those related to safety, effectiveness, and openness. The use of AI in healthcare must be governed by explicit regulations, rigorously test and validate AI algorithms, and hold healthcare providers responsible for adhering to those regulations.

We can make sure that AI is utilized to enhance patient outcomes while preserving the highest standards of safety and effectiveness by solving these regulatory obstacles.

Conclusion

Evaluating the potential benefits and drawbacks of AI in healthcare

By enhancing medical diagnosis and treatments, artificial intelligence (AI) has the potential to transform the healthcare sector. But it also poses serious threats to patients' security, privacy, and general health. It is crucial to consider both the benefits and risks of AI as it is increasingly incorporated into healthcare.

AI has great potential for the healthcare industry. Healthcare professionals may make better judgments because of the rapid and precise analysis of massive volumes of data by AI algorithms. Additionally, this technology can hasten the development of new drugs by detecting diseases at an earlier stage, when they are easier to treat. AI can also enhance the interpretation of medical imaging and assist healthcare professionals in seeing patterns and trends in patient data that would be difficult to find manually.

However, the integration of AI into healthcare also poses significant threats. One of the most serious hazards is prejudice and discrimination, since AI systems may perpetuate and magnify existing biases in healthcare. Additionally, there is the potential for AI algorithms to make mistakes that harm patients. Privacy and security are also key considerations, since AI may pose hazards to the confidentiality and security of patient data.

We must address these issues if we want to make sure that the benefits of AI for healthcare exceed the risks. The use of AI in healthcare must be governed by explicit regulations, rigorously test and validate AI algorithms, and hold healthcare providers responsible for adhering to those regulations. Aside from that, we must make sure AI is applied to medical decision-making in a transparent, ethical, and accountable manner.

In conclusion, although AI has great promise for the healthcare industry, it is important to consider the risks and take precautions against them. We can use the promise of this technology to enhance patient outcomes and advance the science of medicine by tackling the regulatory difficulties and ethical issues related to AI in healthcare.

www.ingramcontent.com/pod-product-compliance
Lightning Source LLC
Chambersburg PA
CBHW070852220526
45466CB00005B/1973